I was sitting at a restaurant when a sharp pain shot out from under my jaw through my ear causing me to jump. After going to the doctor's repeatedly over the next seven months, I was diagnosed with Adenoid Cystic Carcinoma. It started in my salivary gland and had traveled up nerve sheaths. After having a radical neck surgery, I was left with a paralyzed lip and no taste buds on one side of my tongue. I underwent radiation therapy ending up on a feeding tube for months. There is no chemotherapy for this cancer and it metastasized to my lungs four years later. I had half of one of my lungs removed and a portion of the other to cut out four tumors. I am now receiving scans every three months to see where the cancer might show up again. This cancer can be slow growing but is relentless.

The Lord has been good in sending me comfort in times of distress. The Word of God says:

*Blessed be the God and Father of our Lord Jesus Christ, the Father of mercies and God of **all comfort**, who comforts us in **all** our tribulation that we may be able to **comfort those** who are in any trouble, **with the comfort** with which we ourselves are comforted by God. (2 Cor 1:3-5)*

It is my hope that the comfort He has sent me will comfort you in the battle you are fighting. This journey can be quite tumultuous and unpredictable. When we have comfort we are air-bagged in when bumps in the road occur. May the God and Father of our Lord Jesus Christ comfort you in any troubles you may be facing along this road. I pray you will be surrounded by His tender mercies and find great peace in trusting Him.

James 5:13-14

Is anyone among you suffering? Let him pray. Is anyone cheerful? Let him sing psalms. Is anyone among you sick? Let him call for the elders of the church, and let them pray over him, anointing him with oil in the name of the Lord.

Let Them Pray

After a suspicious MRI result, the doctor called me at home and scheduled a needle biopsy for the growth in my neck. The needle biopsy turned out to be inconclusive and a surgical biopsy was scheduled with priority. He called on Tuesday and the surgery was for that Thursday. I had been part of the worship team that

Wednesday and appreciated the opportunity to be with the saints, in His presence and in His Word before such a procedure.

I called for the elders to pray over me and anoint me with oil after church that night. The scriptures are clear that those facing sickness should initiate this. The elders came over to my home after church, sat me in chair in their midst and proceeded to pray for me and anoint me with oil. As I was sitting there, confident I was doing what God had instructed me to do, I heard a voice in my head. I heard two statements. *"Brace for impact." "Are you ready to live what you believe?"* The elders were praying all the requests one would want prayed when facing a biopsy — benign, find nothing, clear it up. But, when I heard these things I knew it was the Lord preparing me for some BIG changes and painful news.

When they finished praying, I told them I was going to pray because this same section of scripture tells the person that is suffering, THEY need to pray. As they kept their hands on me I cried out to the Lord and thanked Him for being a God who is able to prepare us for things we don't even know are coming and that He would grant me the grace to live what I believe.

As we finished I shared what I heard the Lord speak to me and thanked them for praying. There was a somberness in the room but a sense that the Lord was with us and speaking.

We must love the voice of God regardless of what He is speaking. To hear Him gives us a great sense of security in His intimate involvement in our lives. Following His written Word often opens us to His personal spoken Word.

Lord, help me not pick out the verses I want to work in a situation. May I be a person who cares more about hearing Your voice rather than having a preference for what I want You to say. I know that You never sleep or slumber. Your eyes are on me and You might speak to me in a very personal way. I pray I will be quiet enough in my own fears and thoughts to hear You. Speak to me, Lord. Your servant is listening. Be louder than any other voice in my head. When You speak, I am blessed.

Heb 12:1

**...let us run with endurance the race
that is SET before us**

*"I didn't order this. Can I send it
back?"*

When I was diagnosed with cancer I
found myself trying to 'catch up' with
the news. This just wasn't on my short
or long term life-goals list! I went up
to my room, knelt next to my bed and
had a good cry. I needed to release
the shock and dread. I wasn't sure
how to react to all those who were
calling and visiting to share their
concern and pain over my recent
news. As I cried in the presence of the
Lord I heard Him remind me of one of
my earliest prayers as a new believer:

"*Send me Lord WHEREVER You want me to go. Send me where I can be used the most for Your glory and Your purposes.*" In my mind, at that time, I was considering actual locations. Now I realized that He was sending me into "Cancer-land" – a land with its own culture, language and people. This race was SET before me. Now I must RUN it and run it to win for His glory.

Acceptance is one of the first tasks a cancer patient must face. As He reminded me that I did NOT choose this but it was SET before me, I realized that my job now was to RUN it. I was not to drag my feet or try to run away from it, but RUN to win. He would show me how to run it and all I had to do was accept that which was set before me.

Lord, this is NOT the race I wanted to compete in. I thank You that You have prepared me for this more than I realize. Please help me accept the 'new normal' I am experiencing and go beyond acceptance to actually running with it. I know that You go before me and You go with me. May I run with an eagerness to win. Even if I don't win against this disease, I pray for many victories along the way. Comfort me when I am sad. Hold me when I feel alone in this. Give me courage for the difficult. Thank You that You understand my humanity and You will help me gain composure and resolve. In Jesus' name. Amen.

I will lift up my eyes to the hills — From whence comes my help? My help comes from the Lord, Who made heaven and earth.

Where are You Looking?

I went to bed the night I received the cancer diagnosis knowing life as I had been living was just redefined. My husband held me close as we wept together realizing we were now going to be thrust into treatment, surgery and an uncertain amount of days together.

As I slept I had a dream. I was on a beautiful beach as one would see on the east coast. There were wisps of beach grass intermittently standing among the sandy-carpeted terrain. I walked away from the ocean on a wooden board walk and into a two-story beach house. As I entered the house, I saw a wooden oval-shaped carved wall hanging. Carved into it was the scripture reference "Psalm 121:1".

When I woke up I went down stairs to make my teens' lunches. (I found it was very stabilizing to continue in normal day-to-day activities as much as possible). I kept a bible on the kitchen counter so I could write a fresh scripture on their lunch bags each day and pray over them. I looked up Psalm 121:1 and realized the Lord was telling me I was to look UP.

Cancer has a way of making you look all around. We look to doctors, Google, medications, treatments and natural remedies. The Lord was telling me that I was to look UP – THAT was where my help was to come from.

When I was determining which location to have my radiation treatment, we drove out to a facility. When we pulled up to the building, the mountains were clearly visible on the horizon. He even used this verse to direct us to the right place for treatment. Praise Him for His Word and HIS help.

Father, You are above all things. You are on the throne regardless of what may seem daunting or out of control in my life. Lord, there are decisions to be made, perspectives to gain and information to gather. Help me look UP and gain a sense of stability and protection as I see You higher than anything that seems too big for me. This will not happen naturally. I must take the ability to choose that You have given me and intentionally look up to You. I WILL look up. My help comes from You. You might use doctors or medication. You might use a non-conventional method. But, I will look up and know my help comes from You, the Maker of heaven and earth.

Ps 34:8

Oh, taste and see that the Lord is good; Blessed is the man who trusts in Him!

Spiritual Sight and Taste Buds

The cancer I was diagnosed with was in the submandibular gland. This meant that I was facing a radical neck dissection. The doctor told me that he would not know what sort of outcome the surgery would have until he went in and searched for all the cancer. I was informed that I could lose my taste, movement of my shoulder and/or experience permanent facial paralysis. Wow! What news! I went before the Lord and began to pour out my heart. I also realized that this cancer can travel to the lacrimal gland and there was a possibility down the line I could lose an eye. This was overwhelming to me. I might not be able to taste food and not see in the future.   Then,   the   Lord   gently reminded me that I would ALWAYS be able to taste and see HIS goodness. Cancer   would   NEVER   stop   such experiences. It's amazing to me that the earthly trials we go through, no matter HOW painful they may be, can NEVER annul the powerful promises He has given us. When the Lord is our Shepherd we shall lack NOTHING.

Oh Lord, You are aware of the soul-shaking information we often hear in this journey. You are with us when our souls are unsettled. You can give us promises of comfort that address the pain or fears certain news may bring. Thank You that You love us and are deeply concerned about our frame.

You know our frame and You are prepared to undergird us and be the strength of our lives. You often use promises in Your Word to bring comfort and perspective. Your Words are able to address any other words we might hear. May I be in a place of dependence. Help me draw near to You, weep in Your presence and be receptive to the comfort You want to give me.

Ps 91:11

For He shall give His angels charge over you, to keep you in all your ways.

Militant and Positioned

As I was facing a major surgery to remove the tumor and its fingers from my neck, I knew I needed prayer. One day a friend and her companion came up to me and offered to pray for me. Her friend was a bit more expressive in prayer than I was accustomed to. Realizing my doctrinal understanding was competing with my ability to yield and receive, I surrendered my own understanding and placed myself in the care of this gal's passionate and precious prayers. As I positioned myself as one in desperate need of God's touch regardless of how foreign certain approaches to Him might be, I found myself dependent and longing to hear from Him. I had my eyes closed as she was praying over me. Suddenly I began to have a vision. Her words became distant and acted as the soundtrack for this unfolding vision.

I was inside of an operating room. It was empty but prepped for a procedure. The swinging doors to the left abruptly opened and in entered an angelic being. He was crouched down looking to the left and to the right while taking his muscle tissue-like wings and swooping them in a militant and cleansing fashion. He proceeded to move throughout the room sweeping from one side to the other. After completing this mission, he called out something toward the doors. Then entered a small squadron of angelic beings crouching and peering into the room with watchful and attentive glances. They each positioned themselves around the perimeter of the room at equal intervals and assumed a guarded stance with wings drawn together in front of their chests. Once the attending angels took their positions, the lead angel took his place and I could see through the windows the surgical team approaching the swinging doors.

I knew the Lord had given me this vision to let me know that He would commission His warriors on that day. These warrior angels would be in the operating room even though they would not be visible to anyone's eyes. The next morning I was reading a daily devotional and sure enough, the whole reading was about militant, unseen angelic beings. He was assuring me that He truly DOES give His angels charge over us to keep us in all our ways.

Jesus, You are the Captain of the Lord's army. The angelic beings are at Your disposal. Thank You Jesus for showing us that You wept and struggled in the Garden of Gethsemane. You were facing something very difficult and You didn't want to do it. Thank You for showing me it is okay to not like this. Thank You for showing me that I need to be real and honest before God. An angel came to You in that garden and strengthened You. I need strength outside of myself. Send any angels I may need. I trust that there is more support than I recognize. I give You praise and thanks for giving them charge over me to protect me in ALL my ways.

24

Deut 23:5

"...because the Lord your God loves you."

He Loves Us

I had been scheduled to speak at a retreat that was taking place the weekend before my radical neck dissection. Knowing I could immerse myself in His Word, worship and have the precious fellowship of other believers brought me great comfort. This was much needed as I approached such a radical surgery and radiation shortly after. I had accepted the invitation to speak long before my diagnosis. God knew what I was going to face and although I booked it prior to my diagnosis, He most certainly had my good in mind.

I usually drive home on Saturday nights from retreats so I can come alongside my husband in his ministry as he is the senior pastor of our church. He graciously gave me the freedom to stay the entire weekend to be refreshed, encouraged and instructed.

Sunday morning I was sitting in the congregation at this ladies' retreat preparing to receive communion. I sat singing to Him and desiring to receive all He would give me. I longed to give Him all the praise He deserved regardless of my plight. As I was sitting there I heard a scripture reference in my thoughts. I heard, *"Deuteronomy 23:5."* So strange. I never hear references. I am not even really great at remembering the numerical addresses for scriptures. It was loud. It was obvious. I must admit I was a bit scared to look it up. You see, I knew that the book of Deuteronomy was a book that dealt with all kinds of laws and practices God wanted His people to use to govern. Things like; animals falling in ditches, aberrant sexual practices and borrowing thing from each other are in this book. *"What could the Lord say to me in this book? About MY situation right now? How could this reference speak to me about this horrible cancer and all that goes with it,"* I asked myself.

As they handed out the communion, I cautiously opened my bible to see what Deuteronomy 23:5 could POSSIBLY speak to me. I noticed the various ordinances that were written as I searched to reach the exact verse. There, in chapter 23 verse 5, I read:

"Nevertheless the Lord your God would not listen to Balaam, but the Lord your God turned the curse into a blessing for you, because the Lord your God loves you."

In this precious verse the Lord told me He would turn the curse into a blessing. He told me He was going to do this FOR me because the Lord MY

God LOVES me! He was going to take this cancer and turn it into a blessing FOR ME and His motivation was because He LOVES ME!!!! What comfort. What tender words given to me at that moment.

I often held on to this promise and the heart of God I could see behind it throughout the 'cursed' times of this journey. I even 'gave' it to a friend of mine who was greatly distressed at the journey I found myself on. I told her to memorize it and speak it when she felt overwhelmed by the unseen road I was facing.

God's promises are like that. They comfort and confront fears, pain and discouragement. What has He given you?   Ask Him to speak to you and when He does, hold on to His promises throughout those shaky and unfamiliar times you might face.

Lord, You love me. None of this journey should speak anything different to me. You died on the cross for me. THIS is love. Cancer is the result of a fallen world. Our bodies are temporary dwelling places made from the dust and to dust they shall return. But, God, Your love is uninterrupted by the ugly in our lives. I must not interpret Your love for me through this cancer. I will process this cancer through the filter of Your faithful love toward me. Help me hear You and treat Your promises like the valuable commodity they are. In Jesus' name. Amen.

Ps 103:13-14

The Lord is like a father to his children, tender and compassionate to those who fear him. For he knows how weak we are; he remembers we are only dust.

He is Compassionate

When I came home from my surgery I had lost part of my taste buds leaving my tongue burning with neuropathy and a huge scar going across my neck and lockjaw. I felt absolutely trapped in a body I didn't recognize. As I tried to eat I would bite my tongue. Chewing was difficult and since my lower palette had cancer in it, they removed part of it. My tongue could no longer move the food as I had throughout my life. Just trying to eat was overwhelming and unfamiliar. I found myself lost and troubled with my inabilities. I couldn't seem to connect to His presence and my mind was relentlessly plagued with thoughts of weakness and helplessness.

As I walked into the restroom I realized I was not able to sense His leading, His promptings or what He might want from me. Then...I heard His voice. This was the last time I would hear His inner voice for many months due to the rough road that lay ahead during radiation and its effects. He spoke to me, *"I have NO expectations on you."* I knew, at that moment, He was my Father and all He wanted from me was to fight this cancer, get through treatments and recover.

Just as a parent would NOT expect their child to do chores or even speak to them respectfully when they are ill, my Heavenly Father was not looking for anything FROM me. He wanted me to rest and focus on the battle ahead.

Many people projected that the Lord was going to use me with the medical staff and other patients as I was going through treatments. When I heard these forecasts, I was overwhelmed wondering how I could be sensitive to others when I was just trying to chew a small piece of chicken. When the Lord spoke this to me, I knew that I didn't have to DO anything during this season. He was going to take care of ME and He had NO expectations on me.

This gave me peace and the freedom to experience all of the difficult steps ahead without a false expectation of what God was requiring of ME. I could live in the sense that He was taking care of me and I could focus on getting through these tough times without the weight of some preconceived idea of what the Lord was going to do through me. I could rest in His love and trust that this was a season He was not expecting anything FROM me but was going to take good care of me. I was His child. He was my Father. It was my time to rest in His love and care. NO expectations.

When we face such difficult times we must remember that He knows our frame. He knows we are human and we face human things. He is tender and compassionate. Rest in this and take the position as His child, surrendering your fragile frame to His strong and sure care.

Heavenly Father, I thank You that You refer to Yourself as my 'Abba' in Your Word. 'Abba' means 'Daddy'. You know that life can be very hard and You look after us like a daddy looks after his little child when they are scared or in pain. I position myself in Your love, protection and care. Remove from me any preconceived ideas of what You want to do through this journey. May I be at rest knowing You are my Daddy and I am Your child. Thank You for adopting me and calling me Your own. I graciously surrender any expectations I have on myself and take the role of being cared for.

John 13:7

Jesus answered and said to him, "What I am doing you do not understand now, but you will know after this."

You Do Not Understand Now — but You Will

When things come in and want to disrupt our lives it is important that we don't allow them to unnecessarily throw us off course. Sure, there will be changes, but if we seek to be consistent in matters that do NOT have to be interrupted, we will be much more stable in times of uncertainty.

From daily chores to consistent bed times, our lives can run much more smoothly if we seek to be consistent in daily living. Church attendance, daily times with the Lord and serving others help us maintain some order and position us to receive what we might need.

When the biopsy and diagnosis came, I was in the middle of reading a book. As I recovered from the surgical biopsy I sat out on my porch and decided to continue in it. I started right where I left off. The chapter began exploring times when we face things we can't seem to wrap our minds around. We sense that God is in it but really can't begin to understand what He is doing. The author brought me into the scene where Jesus was washing Peter's feet. Peter was aghast! This couldn't possibly be right. The entire scene was not one he could accept or cooperate with.

Jesus was so kind. Jesus told Peter that He knew he didn't understand. He didn't rebuke him for not understanding. Jesus knew by Peter's reaction that Peter did NOT understand. Peter heard his Lord speak to his confusion giving a gentle reminder that *afterward* he would understand. This was not a time of understanding but cooperating.

When we face scenarios that seem confusing and beyond our ability to categorize, it is time to seek the Lord.

We should ask Him for the ability to cooperate rather than challenge. We need His help to accept rather than analyze. We should seek to live life rather than look for logic.

This greatly comforted me. I needed to stop thinking and predicting. I needed to know that it is okay with Jesus that I did NOT understand NOW but later I would.

I am grateful I started that book BEFORE my biopsy and continued reading it after.

What was God using to speak to you before your diagnosis? If possible, get back to those things. You need to hear from Him. Don't let cancer cut you off from the sources of encouragement and truth you need at this time. He will speak to us. We must be in that place to listen.

Jesus, I realize that there are many things I do not understand. Thank you that I do not have to understand. Understanding the reason something happens doesn't necessarily help me go through it. I ask You to forgive me for demanding any sort of explanation. Help me trust You with that which I don't understand. I want to know You better than the details of this journey. Lord, I trust that things will come out of this later and I don't even have to see them. Send me Your comfort and courage. I don't need reasons. Lead me. Guide me. May I fully cooperate without having to understand. In Jesus' name. Amen.

1 Cor 12:4-6

There are diversities of gifts, but the same Spirit. There are differences of ministries, but the same Lord. And there are diversities of activities, but it is the same God who works all in all.

Different Ways to Minister

When I was going through head and neck radiation there were side effects that made life quite unpleasant. One side effect was necrosis. Necrosis is when flesh cells die. Radiation was killing cells in my throat, mouth and nose. Dead flesh produces a rancid odor. I found myself nauseous from the smell and even my husband couldn't kiss or be too close to me because the odor was so bad. Sometimes I would even vomit from the odor. The smell of dead flesh ushered in thoughts of despair and an awareness of the ugliness of this experience.

Different friends were helping me through these rough times. People were cleaning my house, making me meals and stopping by to visit and encourage. A dear friend wanted to help me. She couldn't commit to cleaning. She didn't think cooking was her gift so she prayed. As she prayed she remembered my plight with necrosis. This gal came over with eucalyptus oil and suggested I rub some under my nose to overcome the smell of death. Upon doing this, the sweet smell of eucalyptus conquered the bitter odor of decaying flesh. No more nausea. No more vomiting. My husband could, once again, hold me near to give me comfort.

God uses different people for different sources of comfort. Be open to receiving and giving comfort in non-predictable ways. When we pray and ask God to send us comfort or use us to comfort others, we position ourselves to be receptive to His creative leading. We must not compare one person's act of love with another's. Each is unique and each is helpful. Let us remain open and available to what the Lord wants to do uniquely through us and for us.

Lord, I believe You want to comfort people. You use people. Help me be open to people and the different ways they might want to help me during this journey. Help me appreciate their help and soak in the love they are seeking to show me. Help me lower my expectations on others. May I be humble to ask for help when I need it and be thankful when others do. May I recognize Your love flowing through others and allow them to be vessels of support and strength. Send those You know I need. In Jesus' name. Amen.

Ps 119:105

Your word is a lamp to my feet And a light to my path.

His Word Counsels Us

I was steadily losing weight as I could no longer eat any food due to side effects of head and neck radiation. My throat had ulcers, all of my taste buds were gone and swallowing was painful and difficult to do. My doctor had told me that it was up to me to make the decision of whether to have a gastronomy feeding tube (G-tube) surgically placed in order to receive liquid nutrition directly into my stomach.

My husband was concerned about hydration and my consistent weight loss but was hesitant to encourage me to get the G-tube. The doctor spoke to us about this option but the decision was ours. My husband looked at the G-tube as a drastic measure. We left the office to drive home.

That day, a dear friend, had driven us the long distance to radiation and asked us how we would know whether we should choose the G-tube. I told her that we would pray, seek the Lord for leading and look to the Word of God for counsel. She wondered how the written Word of God could give us such direction on a medical matter.

We got home and I took up my regular place on the double recliner in my room, weak and starving. A friend was over and offered to read the Word of God to me. He proceeded to read from the place he was reading in his daily time with the Lord.

Dare any of you, having a matter against another, go to law before the unrighteous, and not before the saints? (1 Cor 6:1)

As much as I love the Word of God, this particular verse didn't seem to comfort me in my cancer affliction. I reminded myself that all scripture is breathed by God and can profit us in some way. Sitting there listening, I believed that hearing God's voice can be just as calming as the words He may speak to us. Then, my friend read this verse in 1 Cor 6:13, "*Foods for the stomach and the stomach for foods...*" My husband, who was resting on the bed, sat up immediately and my eyes opened wide. We believed we had just received direction from the written word of God about placing the G-tube in my stomach so I could get nutrition. This verse tied food straight to the stomach without going through the mouth and throat. What a wonderful surprise and yet such clear, calming counsel. We knew, at that moment, God was leading us to go through the procedure for me to get the food I needed.

In context, this verse has nothing to do with a G-tube. To force scriptures to speak to us about contemporary issues can be inappropriate and reckless. But, if the Holy Spirit chooses to illuminate a verse and speak to us in such a way, it is His decision because the bible is the Sword of the Spirit.

This experience touched my heart that my Father would take His Word and direct it to me to give me light for my path. It is important for us to stay in the written Word of God knowing He sends His Word to us to instruct, lead and reveal.

Lord, You want to guide us. You are a Shepherd and we are Your sheep. Shepherds lead their sheep. It is who You are. I can trust that You will lead me. You can use Your written Word, others' advice, inner peace, a sense of restraint and countless other ways to lead me. May I approach each decision of this battle seeking You to lead me. You know what is best for me. Help me to gather facts I need and ignore those I don't. Above all, let me sense Your will for my life.

Ps 34:1

I will bless the Lord at all times; His praise shall continually be in my mouth.

At ALL Times

I had just returned from the bathroom having vomited up what little contents were in my stomach. My throat was inflamed from radiation and the gag reflex was in full effect. If I spoke or swallowed incorrectly, I would vomit although I had no nausea. I chose not to talk for a few weeks to avoid dehydration and unnecessary loss of nutrition.

As I sat on the side of my bed I was weary and the quality of my life seemed to be getting worse with every passing day. Another 'normal' life activity had been erased from my life. Now I could not have verbal connection with those around me. This new chapter left me emotionally depleted and weary.

At that moment I could hear the taunting of my adversary. A distant voice challenged the faithfulness and the love of God. The enemy was speaking mocking criticisms of my God using my weak and weary condition as evidence of God's lack of love for me.

I couldn't perceive God's presence with me. All of the pain and problems were louder and more obvious than His voice and presence. At that moment, I remembered the cross and the restored relationship Christ had given me through His sacrifice. I KNEW God was for me because of what Christ had done for me before I even existed. His love for me was not wrapped up in what was happening to me now. His love was evidenced by what He had already done for me. I could not feel His presence with me but I knew He was with me. He didn't have to do ONE more thing for me. His great sacrifice for my sins demonstrated His love to me and nothing in this temporary life could sabotage such a selfless and thorough act of love for me!

As tears flowed down my face, I whispered softly and yet firmly without gagging, *"Your praise will continually be on my lips."* I would praise Him in the midst of ugly and hard times because I didn't need Him to do anything more to prove His love for me. He was faithful and He loved me. Jesus gave it all for me. I was loved.

Lord Jesus, thank You for going to the cross for me. Thank You for loving me before I was even created. Thank You for demonstrating Your love for me by Your sacrifice on Calvary. I will be confident in Your love for me because of what HAS been done. You said it was finished when You breathed Your last breath on this earth. Father, if You did not hold back Your own Son, how can I doubt that You will hold back anything I need now. I will praise You for who You are and not allow the enemy's lies to define who You are to me.

Ps 116:9

I will walk before the Lord In the land of the living.

Live

Being diagnosed with cancer can be quite daunting. The awareness that someone has moved into your body and you didn't put out a *'room for rent'* sign can make you feel violated and victimized. I felt like there was a tenant living in my body I wanted to evict but couldn't.

The Lord began to show me through this allegory about the cancer. Just as if a person were living in my home that I didn't want living there, I could adapt to this roommate as well. If someone occupied a room in my house and were smelly, messy or unwelcomed, there would still be the rest of my home I could keep clean, enjoy and live in. I wouldn't have to give that one member of the household the ability to define the entire state of my home.

I realized that there was SO much more to my life than the cancer. I was responsible for the areas I *did* have influence over. I could exercise, enjoy good food and friends. I could get my hair done, play with my dog and invest in my family. I could pray with others, take in a sunset and travel for now. Cancer would affect me but I refused to let it define me.

It is important we understand that although cancer will change our lives, we must intentionally position ourselves in the land of the living. We are not dead. We are alive.

I must live. I am not dead. I have this moment. I have this day. Lord, You want me to believe that I will see Your goodness in the land of the living. Help me to live and not just exist. Help me experience all the beauty around me. Help me love people and even if I am having a difficult time connecting, help me immerse myself in healthy relationships. Lord, put me where I need to be. May I not give in to my feelings but yield to You and Your leading in my life. Lord, may this cancer not upstage all the other wonderful things You have blessed me with. In Jesus' name. Amen.

Eccl 4:12

Though one may be overpowered by another, two can withstand him.

They Understand

I had recently received bad news from my routine CT-scan. There were tumors in my lungs. Now the cancer moved to stage four – metastatic cancer. This meant the cancer had entered either my vascular or lymphatic system; it had invaded my body.

This was sad news. Our family vacation was already scheduled and we left to Santa Barbara shortly after receiving the report. As we were on the trip I found myself trying to catch up with this information. I knew this was big. I was no longer waiting to see if cancer had come back. It was there and moved into other parts of my body.

I knew I had to process this information and accept my new normal. I needed to work through and adjust to being 'terminal.'

My family is precious and understanding, but I knew this was not going to be something I wanted to dialogue with them about. It was deep. It was personal. It shook me to the core. I needed another human to join with me in this experience but it was much too weighty to put on my family.

I began to search my electronic book device for someone else's terminal illness story. After looking through a few that were not rooted in the hope of Christ, I found a self-published book by a believer who was facing multiple sclerosis.

I read through his story in a few hours. There were a few tidbits that jumped out to me but mainly I had fellowship in my sufferings. He was further down the road than I was, and his perspective helped me orient myself in this new land.

It is important to connect with others who have faced or are facing similar experiences. The Lord knows that two are better than one. When one falls down, the other can lift them up. When we feel isolated we may implode and are much more susceptible to the enemy's lies and attacks on God's character. Being connected to like-minded people can produce resiliency and fight within.

Check out books, testimonies or videos of others that have walked your path. Even if your experiences vary it is always comforting to know that others are travelling difficult roads as well.

Father bring people across my path that would be good to relate to. Show me any support groups, on-line connections, books or other resources that could bring me encouragement. Use me to come alongside someone in this journey. Help me not isolate myself but be willing to connect with others in similar suffering. Thank You that You said 'Two are better than one." I trust You and will accept this truth knowing You are right.

Phil 4:8

"...whatever things are lovely, whatever things are of good report...If there is anything praiseworthy — meditate on these things."

What CAN You Do?

Friends came over to visit me after my major neck surgery. A dear family came to visit and show their love and support.

As I sat on the couch they asked me to tell them what the repercussions of the surgery were. The cancer had eaten many nerves so they had to be surgically removed. I began to tell them about the taste buds being gone, paralyzed lip, my tongue having restricted movement, removal of salivary glands resulting in dry mouth and the numbness of my tongue.

One of their little girls was listening with quite the focus. After I was finished sharing all I couldn't do now as a result of the surgery, she got my attention.

"*Mrs. Schaffer,*" she spoke. I looked at her and asked her what she would like to say. She stood up in the middle of all of us. She began to wave each arm and each leg one after another while saying, "*You can do this and you can do that and you can do this and you can do that!*"

What a glorious truth! She demonstrated all I COULD do. It was a great perspective in the midst of my new normal. She taught me to look at ALL I COULD do. What a gift she was to me that day and what a gift her insight is still.

Sometimes when I feel restricted or overwhelmed by changes as a result of the cancer, I imitate her. I stand up and shake my right arm saying, "*I can do this.*" Then, I shake my left arm and say, "*I can do that.*" I shake my right leg and say, "*I can do this.*" Then, I shake my left leg and say, "*I can do that!*"

That precious little girl taught me that we must always balance our losses with what we DO have. We will avoid exaggerating our losses by focusing on what we CAN do.

Oh Lord, You know the changes I am facing and You want to give me a good perspective. There are so many restrictions because of this cancer that I can feel like I am missing out on life. Open my eyes to see what I CAN do. Let me be a grateful person. I will verbally give thanks to You. This will help me silence the self-pity that can beat me down. Lord, magnify the health I still have and help me use my health in ways that glorify You and keep me living.

Dan 2:28

"But there is a God in heaven who reveals secrets"

Revealer of Secrets

Cancer is something that is not usually diagnosed until certain tests reveal its presence. Scans, blood work and pathology are used to see things we cannot see with the naked eye.

When we are waiting for results of a scan we can be very anxious. This time of worry has been appropriately nicknamed "scan-xiety". The phone rings and we could receive news we may have feared.

These times can be very hard. But, our God is the One who reveals secrets.

He knows if there are any cancer cells and where they are. Knowing this, we can rest that He has the results of any scan and is actively involved in preparing us for the news.

The unknown can be frightening but when we know God knows, we can curl up next to Him. We can thank Him for knowing. We can trust He will be with us when the secrets are revealed. We mustn't be afraid to know. Knowing will help us fight the cancer.

Light is good. God wants to bring things to the light so we walk in truth. He is the revealer of secrets. He may use a machine, doctor or pathologist. Let's calm our restless hearts and during the waiting time, take courage realizing that He knows and He reveals.

Lord, the unknown can scare me. I thank You that You see all things. The technology that enables my doctors to see things, exists because You wove those engineering truths into Your creation. When I am waiting for results, help me have peace knowing You already know. Lord, lead my health care providers to discover all they need to, in order to give me the best care. Hide false positives and reveal anything that needs to be seen. Help me pray through the procedures and know You see all. I can trust in You while I wait. If I do, I will renew my strength rather than be depleted.

John 14:27-28

Peace I leave with you, My peace I give to you; not as the world gives do I give to you. Let not your heart be troubled, neither let it be afraid.

Shalom

My doctor was researching whether the tumors in my lung could be surgically removed. I did the 'Google' research myself. After reading many worst-case scenarios I found myself a bit apprehensive about having my lungs violated with a surgeon's knife. Would I wake up from surgery gasping for air? Would my quality of life be greatly diminished? What would another 'new normal' be like?

I attended a women's retreat while waiting for the decision. During a time of worship I began to bring my concerns before the Lord. As I sang to Him I poured out my cares and cast my anxieties upon Him. When I exalt Him and bring my concerns before Him simultaneously, I find myself much more secure than when I just bring those things to Him without praise. I brought my concern about waking up in post-op having had my lungs cut open. I told Him how concerned I was with the initial waking up from anesthesia and coming to grips with the outcome. As I was praising/praying I heard His still, small voice speak within my mind. *"If you have the surgery, peace will meet you."* I heard His voice! What a joy! What relief!

The peace He spoke of was not a feeling or sense of calm. He communicated this peace was going to be a companion to me. This peace was going to be personified, as if a friend was greeting me as I awoke from the surgery. I was amazed at how He made it so clear. He had assured me that peace would meet me in that post-op bay. Tears fell from my eyes. I knew that I was not to visit that fear again. The Lord would send peace to meet me if I ended up having the surgery.

A few months later I was scheduled for the first of two lung surgeries. I had shared the precious Word the Lord gave me with my husband and a few friends. I held on to this as the day approached for the surgery.

They brought me in on a Sunday morning when no other patients were scheduled. It was quiet and peaceful in the waiting area. No one was manning the front desk as the surgical unit was normally closed on Sundays. My family waited with me in the waiting room. My daughter had flown in from Arizona to be with me. I hadn't told her about 'peace' meeting me. Soon, they would come to the door and call my name. I would go into that pre-op/post-op area.

My daughter asked the name of my thoracic surgeon. When I told her his name she said that his name sounded Jewish. I told her I thought he was. She said, "*You know what that means, mom?*" I answered her with, "*No, what does that mean?*"

"*That means Shalom is waiting to meet you in there!*"

My husband and I were in shock! I asked her if she had heard about what the Lord told me a few months ago. She assured me she hadn't. What a confirmation! Shalom is the Hebrew word for 'peace'. I was absolutely comforted by her words. Now I faced the procedure doubly spoken that truly peace/shalom would meet me in there.

The nurse came to the door and called my name. My husband and I got up to go back and begin down this road. I was not worried. Peace/shalom would meet me there. The nurse checked my band as we walked through the door. She then introduced herself, *"Hello, I will be your nurse, my name is Shalom."* Yes. You read that correctly! The nurse's name was SHALOM!!!!!!! My husband and I froze in our paths. What an incredible evidence of God's personal involvement in my life. Tears of joy and a great sense of God's tender mercies flooded our hearts.

Our God is greatly concerned with our concerns. He knows when we need evidences of His great love. The greatest evidence of His love for us is in sending His Son to die and receive the punishment we deserved.

"...this is love...He loved us and sent His Son to be the propitiation for our sins." (1 Jn. 4:10-11)

When we choose to yield to Him as our God, exalting Him and casting our cares on Him, He will sustain us. We must realize that He loves us more than we could possibly perceive. He promises to be with us in troubles. He knows when we are fearful and as any good Father would do, will send comfort.

Lord, help us to come to you with our fears and concerns. May we exalt you and praise you in times of anxiety. May we be quiet enough to hear Your voice. Send Your comfort to us. Help us to be confident in your care.

Ps 105:1

Oh, give thanks to the Lord!

Go Beyond the Moment

There is a mask one wears when receiving head and neck radiation. It is form-fitted to your face and bolted into the board you lay on so that the radiation is directed away from healthy tissue in the head and neck area. It is difficult to even blink because it is so tight. They don't want you to be able to slightly move. It can be a bit claustrophobic.

After the technicians bolt you down, they leave you alone in the room. They know that radiation is dangerous and as they close the large metal door you are left with a red light glowing and a machine that moves around you, shooting radiation into your body hoping to kill any newly forming cancer cells.

This experience can be quite daunting. The seriousness of your illness confronts you and you realize that this is a life and death fight. It is not pleasant and with every session new symptoms appear. I ended up with mouth ulcers, throat ulcers and lost the ability to eat. A gastric tube was put in my stomach and liquid nutrition sustained me. I didn't like radiation at all!

A couple of things helped me through the 30 sessions of radiation therapy. I brought worship music into the room to listen to as I was going through the process. This music reminded me that I am to praise the Lord at ALL times. No matter how ugly things are, He is STILL beautiful!

Another thing that helped me was to begin the session giving thanks to the Lord. I thanked Him that they had found the cancer and we were battling it. It no longer lurked undetected and unrestrained. I thanked Him for the science behind the MRI's and the radiation machine. I thanked Him for the health insurance we had. I thanked Him that my husband was outside the facility in the garden interceding for me. As I thanked Him, I found myself accepting where I was.

I was able to receive the treatment with gratitude even though I didn't like it.

I also spent the rest of the time praying for a mission work in South Africa. This was my commitment. All 30 sessions would be used to intercede for the church there in Johannesburg. You see, Johannesburg was REALLY far away and this helped me travel to a distant land while locked in this basement vault. I knew I was accomplishing great things while bolted to a board. The gates of hell cannot stand against the church. Cancer would not either. This helped me look beyond the momentary unpleasantness and be a part of something bigger.

Lord, show me what would help me in difficult experiences in this cancer journey. Help me cooperate with your suggestions and trust Your advice is good for me.

1 Chron 17:11

And it shall be, when your days are fulfilled, when you must go to be with your fathers...

Our Days Have a Max

We may feel like our days are being cut short by cancer. This is NOT true. The Lord is telling Hezekiah about his death.   The Lord uses the phrase, "when your days are fulfilled." We will not leave this earth until our days are fulfilled. We don't' need to mourn the events we might not attend or grandchildren we might never meet as if we were supposed to be there.   If we die before these things happen, our days were fulfilled.   We reached our max.

Years ago, people would die from even a small open wound. Antibiotics were not available, plagues ran rampant and death in childbirth was a common thing. We are blessed to have such great medical advances and many of us would have died long before the cancer if we had been born in a different time.

We can shed tears for those we leave behind and the change of landscape our absence might bring, but we must not think God is cutting our lives short if we die from the cancer. Our times are in His hands. If we leave, our days are fulfilled.

Lord, I pray you will help us not be afraid to die. Jesus, you set us free from the slavery of being afraid to die when you conquered death. You rose from the dead and promise that in Christ we will be made alive again. Lord, if we are human we will die. If we are Yours we will rise again. Thank you for that promise. May it bring us peace and save us from unnecessary pain and mourning.

If you want to be assured that when your body no longer works, the real you will be with the Lord pray this prayer. If you mean it, you can be assured that even death itself has no final power over you:

Lord Jesus, I believe you died for MY sins. Thank you for taking the punishment I deserve for my sin. You rose from the dead proving that sin was paid for. The wages of sin is death but the gift of God is eternal life. I know what I deserve and I thank You for taking it upon Yourself to suffer for me. Thank You that You want me reconciled to You. Be my Lord. Be my Savior. I surrender my life to You. You will be my guide even to death.

53500339R00054

Made in the USA
San Bernardino, CA
19 September 2017